-75 LBS LATER:
FITNESS AND NUTRITION GUIDE

Table of Contents

INTRODUCTION

A healthy weight is not about following a diet or program. Instead, it involves a lifestyle with healthy eating patterns, regular physical activity, and stress management. Compared to people who lose weight quickly, those who lose gradually and steadily—roughly one to two pounds per week—are more likely to keep the weight off. In addition, sleep, ageing, heredity, illnesses, drugs, and surroundings can all have an impact on weight management.

Setting realistic and achievable goals to overcome weight loss challenges, developing a healthy eating plan and regular exercise program, and maintaining a positive attitude and constant motivation are essential. It is also helpful to seek support from friends, family or a health professional and avoid falling into restrictive diets or extreme eating habits that may be unsustainable in the long term.

It can be understood how discouraging it can be to diet and exercise for years with unsatisfactory weight loss results. Sometimes, you feel like fighting an uphill battle or even going backwards. Due to social pressure and life's demands and expectations, the path to weight loss can be isolating, confusing, and downright impossible. And with new fad diets and pills being advertised more every day, it's getting harder and harder to know what's best for your body.

That's why this book offers a variety of weight loss solutions tailored to your needs. We have monitored this transformation because it is possible to reach a healthy weight and maintain it long-term. When you start with a foundation of healthy eating and physical activity, the foundation for success is laid. If an additional procedure or prescription is necessary to achieve your desired results, we help you achieve it.

Earning a "Before and After" moment of weight loss – whether a sensation or a pose captured in a photo – is the pride of a job well done. It's your satisfaction when you commit to the journey and allow the right help. We conquer weight loss together, step by step.

When it comes to fitness and nutrition, there is no one-size-fits-all-all. This truth is especially evident when looking at protein requirements for women. Breaking free from outdated stereotypes, we're here to demystify women's unique protein needs on their fitness journey. The world of fitness and sports is fascinating, but to attain your goals, you must eat appropriately. If you are a woman looking to maximize her performance and recovery before and after training, you are in the right place.

Say goodbye to misconceptions and hello to science-backed knowledge that allows you to achieve your health and fitness goals effectively.

CHAPTER ONE

Mind Transformation: "I don't know where to start"

Building a Positive Mindset

Mindset is a fundamental aspect of success in any area of life. It is essential to understand that mindset is not innate but develops over time and practice. Some people have a positive mindset from the start, while others may need to work harder to develop it.

Positive mindset is based on the belief that our actions, thoughts and emotions can influence our experiences and outcomes. Through a positive mindset, we can change our perspective and focus, allowing us to overcome challenges with resilience and stay focused on our goals.

The importance of a positive mindset

Below are some key benefits of developing a positive mindset personally and professionally:

1. **Better health and well-being:** A positive mindset is associated with better physical and emotional health. Studies have shown that optimistic people have more robust immune systems, less stress, and greater longevity. Additionally, a positive mindset helps us manage stress more effectively and have a more remarkable ability to recover from difficulties.

2. **Greater resilience:** A positive mindset allows us to face challenges with resilience and perseverance. Instead of collapsing in the face of obstacles, we adopt a learning attitude and look for creative solutions. Resilience helps us overcome

failures and remain steadfast in pursuing our goals.

3. **Better performance:** Positive mindset is related to higher performance in various areas of life. Focusing on possibilities and what we can achieve makes us more motivated and committed to our tasks. Additionally, a positive mindset allows us to learn from mistakes and constantly seek improvement and growth.

Strategies to develop a positive mindset

This article will discuss strategies to develop a positive mindset and achieve success. The following are some practical tips to build a positive mindset. We will also discover how exercise and playing sports can strengthen our positive mindset.

1. Practice self-care:

Taking care of oneself is crucial to keeping an optimistic outlook. Spend time engaging in enjoyable and stress-relieving activities, such as reading a book, relaxing, or engaging in your favorite hobby. Maintaining your mental and physical health will make it easier to deal with obstacles constructively.

It's imperative to return to fundamentals like healthy eating and sleeping. Be mindful of the people, places, and even media that you allow in your life. You feel better and find it easier to keep a positive outlook when caring for yourself.

2. Practice positive visualization:

Positive visualization is a powerful technique that allows you to imagine and experience positive situations mentally. Please spend a few minutes each day visualizing your goals and objectives and envisioning yourself accomplishing them.

Visualization is an effective tool for cultivating a positive mindset. Visualize your success and how it feels to reach your objectives. Consider every detail of what you are attempting to accomplish. Visualization assists you in focusing on your goals and motivating yourself to achieve them.

3. Develop positive affirmations:

Positive affirmations are powerful statements that help us change our self-talk and strengthen our positive mindset. Create affirmations that reinforce your strengths and propel you toward success. Repeat them daily, especially in times of doubt or adversity. For example, "I am capable of overcoming any obstacle" or "I am worthy of love and happiness."

Identify your limiting beliefs and work on transforming them into more positive and empowering beliefs. Visualize your goals and repeat positive affirmations reinforcing your confidence in yourself and your abilities.

4. Learn to control your thoughts:

Our thoughts have a significant impact on our mentality. If you find yourself stuck in negative thought patterns, learning to control them is crucial. The first thing you should do is identify your negative thoughts. It can be challenging initially since negative thoughts often develop habits and become automatic. However, as you begin to pay attention to your thoughts, you will notice how many are hostile and self-destructive.

When you find yourself thinking about something negative, stop and ask yourself why you are thinking it. Is there any evidence to support that thought, or is it just a guess? How does that thought make you feel? Is it helping you achieve your goals or is it holding you back?

Take time to reflect on your thoughts and emotions. Identify negative patterns and work on replacing them with more positive and constructive thoughts. Self-reflection will help you become aware of your thoughts and consciously change them.

5. Learn from your mistakes

Everybody makes mistakes because nobody is flawless. Take lessons from your mistakes rather than letting them define you. Examine what went wrong and decide how to improve things next time. Keep in mind that failures present chances for development.

6. Adopt an attitude of gratitude

Developing an optimistic outlook can be greatly aided by practicing gratitude. Make time each day to reflect on your blessings. You can simply make a mental list or maintain a gratitude notebook. If you focus on the positive, you will learn to appreciate the blessings around you and find joy in the little things in life.

Gratitude is one of the most effective tools for developing a positive mindset. By focusing on the things you have and appreciating them, you shift your focus from the negative to the positive. Start practicing gratitude daily; list what you are grateful for and focus on them. It can be as simple as having a roof over your head or having a hot meal on your table.

7. Surround yourself with positive people

The environment you are in can influence your mindset. Surround yourself with positive and motivating people who inspire and support you on your path to developing a positive mindset. Share your goals and challenges with them; together, you can propel yourself to success.

The people you spend time with have a significant influence on your mindset. If you spend time with negative people, you are more likely to adopt their way of thinking. Therefore, it is vital to surround yourself with positive people who support and encourage you to achieve your goals. Find people who make you feel good and who inspire you.

8. Honor your accomplishments.

Make sure to celebrate your accomplishments when they come to pass. Acknowledge and commemorate your successes, no matter how minor. It supports your motivation to keep going after your objectives.

9. Find inspiration in exercise and sports:

Exercise and playing sports not only benefit our body but also our mind. Physical activity releases endorphins, known as the "happy hormones," which make us feel good and elevate our mood. Additionally, exercise challenges us, helps us set goals, and provides us with a sense of achievement and self-improvement, thus strengthening our positive mindset.

In conclusion, a positive mindset is a powerful tool to boost personal and professional growth. Through a positive mindset, we can face challenges with resilience, stay motivated, and maximize our opportunities. By developing a positive mindset, we open the door to possibilities and become creators of our success. Be patient with yourself and keep at it; a positive mindset comes from practice. You can achieve success with ease!

CHAPTER TWO

Creative Healthy Eating: "Salad tastes like air."

What is healthy eating? Eat a good variety of natural foods (nothing or minimally processed) without excesses, prioritizing those of plant origin. And without forgetting physical exercise. While allowing for occasional indulgences, eating a healthy, balanced diet should be the general rule in our daily lives.

It's something easy to say but not always easy to do; Obligations and fast paces of life can kill creativity or leave us with almost no time to cook. Having a good repertoire of recipes for healthy eating can get us out of a lot of trouble with weekly menus and recipes for weight loss.

The times you eat, the number of dishes you eat daily, and the ingredients you choose are some of the critical pieces for a nutritious, healthy, complete diet. It is through food that you receive the nutrients, vitamins, proteins, minerals and other substances necessary for the proper functioning of your body. Thus, food has a direct relationship with your well-being and health.

The time is now to start adopting a healthier lifestyle and modifying unhealthy eating habits that may affect your health. It is vital to set clear and achievable healthy eating goals to do this. Maintaining a healthy diet is one of the fundamental measures to prevent diseases such as diabetes, hypertension or heart disease and guarantee a healthier old age. Embrace creative food as a fun way to fuel, facilitate and enjoy your nutrition.

Here are some guidelines so that you are encouraged to put creative eating into practice step by step until it becomes a healthy habit.

These are some of the objectives to achieve healthy eating:

1. Prepare weekly menus to facilitate the purchase and preparation of food and ensure the variety and quality of food. Remember the five feeding moments in the day. Discover new foods and more freshness with local vegetables and fruits that are in the harvest season. Dare to use the Menu Planner, a tool that allows you to program your weekly diet, guaranteeing flavor, variety and nutrition.

2. Incorporate fruits and vegetables into your meals: Consuming five servings of fruits and vegetables per day is advised. Try to consume five servings of fresh fruits and vegetables each day.

3. They have essential micronutrients for the body's functioning such as iron, vitamins A, B complex, C and folic acid. Its micronutrients have antioxidant action that promotes cell regeneration. Include them as part of your creative meal by cutting them into geometric and unexpected shapes, think about them when you feel hungry and explore all their textures and colors to eat them in different flavors every day at every moment. Sometimes, it is not easy to start including them in your diet, but a recommendation is to set the goal of consuming two or three servings a day, and after achieving this first goal, increase the portions. Apart from their nutritional value, which includes high levels of vitamins, proteins, and iron, a diverse array of fruits and vegetables can create many delectable dishes.

4. Every day, you can consume an egg and a portion of dairy food: milk, cheese, yoghurt, or kumis because they contain proteins and calcium, nutrients that

promote the health of your muscles, bones and teeth.

5. Complement your diet with legumes and legumes such as beans, lentils, peas and chickpeas at least twice a week. They provide protein, which helps the growth and maintenance of muscles; vitamins that help vision, skin hydration, the transmission of nerve impulses, hair and nail integrity; and strengthen the immune system's defenses. There are numerous recipes to enjoy in soups, creams, hummus, and croquettes of different colors. Dare to change the recipes!

6. Reduce the consumption of processed products: packaged potatoes, boxed juices, cakes with high-added sugar and saturated fats should be consumed as little as possible. They can be replaced by foods such as whole grains, nuts and grains that contain a high fiber content, which is extremely important to include in our diet.

7. Look for healthier preparation alternatives: make more steamed and grilled preparations and look for other ways of cooking that do not involve immersion in oil such as the air fryer. These alternatives will allow us to eat healthier and reduce the amount of fried foods consumed weekly.

8. Hydrate with water and not with fruit juice: the problem with drinking these juices is that when blending the fruit, a high fiber content is lost and in its place, high levels of sugar remain, as in the case of orange juice that contains a high glycemic index. According to this, our drink of choice should be water, which has many health benefits, considering the restrictions on water intake for patients with diseases such as heart failure.

9. Limit your salt intake to protect your blood pressure and heart health. You can use

various techniques in your inventive cooking, such as learning how to cook with less salt, clearing the table of the salt shaker, and seasoning and flavoring food with herbs, spices, lemon, and other flavors that are pure in color and scent.

10. Accompany diet with physical activity: A healthy diet must be combined with physical exercise to create a lifestyle. The preceding includes not just prescribed exercise but also an enjoyable activity that corresponds to each person's physical state. Jogging in a park, dancing or using the machines in public parks are alternatives to start doing physical activity and increase the intensity over time. In addition to scheduled exercise, it is essential to stay active in our daily routine, not sit for more than two hours working, and if some type of short trip is required, walk instead of using transportation to increase the movement level.

11. Have the help of a specialist: the guidance of a nutritionist is crucial and essential for people who are overweight or obese. These must have a guided and personalized process through a healthy eating plan coupled with physical activity. Honesty in this type of process is crucial to guarantee success.

One of the recommendations to achieve these objectives is to understand that a dietary change is not immediate but rather involves a conscious process and evaluation of progress. It is necessary to be realistic with oneself and recognize that there will be failures along the way; however, the secret is not to give up on the goal and to recognize that what we do most of the time counts more in achieving it.

CHAPTER THREE

Effective Workouts: "I can't do push-ups."

Adaptation is responsible for improving sports performance. At a biological level, it represents the reorganization of a biological system by shifting its operating limits. Adaptation is the set of modifications given in a biological system as a consequence of a change in external or internal conditions. At the training level, adaptation is the modification of the athlete's functional systems caused by the stimulus of physical exercise and that seeks to adapt functional capacities to the loads applied at work.

When we talk about adaptation, we mean adapting the organism's capabilities to the workloads. This aspect is fundamental because it is associated with each person's functional and structural transformations. Exercise and physical activity generate a variety of alterations in the body, such as morphological changes, functional and metabolic modifications, and improvements in the coordination of the regulatory activities of the nervous and hormonal systems. Therefore, when doing any exercise, it is necessary to keep in mind that these bring health benefits. Still, they may also have contraindications if an adequate adaptation process is not carried out.

Below are the benefits and contraindications that exercise may have in relation to the adaptation process:

1. The body is better prepared at the respiratory level since it manages oxygen more efficiently, thus giving more excellent help to all other organs to perform their functions optimally.

2. It improves the use of glucose by using it as energy. In addition, it delays ageing since growth hormone is stimulated.

3. It Produces an improvement in intermuscular coordination (greater coordination and quality of movement.)

4. It keeps the brain healthy and releases hormones such as endorphins, which produce a feeling of well-being; serotonin, which improves mood and sleep; and adrenaline which regulates heart rate.

5. Increases the exercise threshold for established symptoms or signs of diseases such as angina pectoris, ST-segment ischemia, and claudication.

With the new panorama we are experiencing thanks to COVID-19, training at home has become part of many people's daily routines and is undoubtedly a way to stay healthy and improve physically. However, doing it autonomously or only with information on the Internet and social networks can make the training design not inadequate due to a lack of knowledge about adaptability to individual capabilities. You need to choose the training well and know how to adjust it to your own physical conditions.

That is why it is crucial to know, from a self-care perspective, how adaptation makes the body improve noticeably and comprehensively. Before starting a workout, you should ask yourself:

- How is your health?

- What exercises you could do and which ones you couldn't?

- Do you have any medical restrictions?

- If so, how does this restriction affect you concerning physical exercise?

These types of questions are essential. If you have doubts about any of them, it is always best to consult first with the appropriate medical personnel before doing any physical activity.

If you have no doubts about your state of health, wonderful! You can start with your high-intensity training, but wait a minute! You must prepare your body, and the best way to start is with an excellent general physical adaptation until you achieve an adequate muscular and cardiovascular base. Below are some recommendations:

1. Choose physical activities that motivate you and make you feel fulfilled in the process. It begins with physical exercise progressively, emphasizing aerobic resistance to adapt all organs and systems, allowing the body to properly assimilate the physical stress that occurs in the practice of exercise. Some examples are skipping jumping jack and aerobic rumba classes.

2. When you adapt to aerobic exercises, begin muscle strengthening with activities with your weight. I will help you prevent injuries in the adaptation process—for example, chair dips, chair squats, push-ups and sit-ups.

3. When planning training, whether autonomously or directed by experts, it is usual to start with an adaptation period that emphasizes the aerobic base and leaves high-intensity work for later.

4. Workouts are favorable but also very demanding due to the intensity of work, which is why prior adaptation is so important. Once the body has developed better strength, endurance, speed and flexibility capabilities, it can do this type of training

safely and efficiently without causing physiological or biomechanical problems, avoiding any type of risk and maintaining good body balance.

A well-oriented adaptation process generates adequate functioning in the cardiovascular and musculoskeletal systems, allowing a consequent improvement in the physical capacity of people.

Although every training session must always be individualized, a series of points of the general structure must be met. These are especially important in cardiological patients to avoid health risks and prevent possible injuries.

1. Warm-up phase

All training sessions should begin with a first warm-up phase. It is recommended that its duration be approximately 10-15 minutes and that it consist of three fundamental parts that are set out below and that must be completed in this order:

- Joint mobility

- Cardiorespiratory activation

- Large muscle group stretches

2. Exercise phase

In this phase, the prescribed training will be carried out, which will be predominantly aerobic in the case of cardiovascular patients, normally walking, running or cycling for specific resistance work. Don't worry if you can only do 10-15 minutes of exercise initially, the important thing is that you progress over time.

The final objective is to gradually progress in this phase until you can maintain 45 minutes to 1 hour of resistance along with increasing the intensity of the session (always complying with your doctor's individualized prescription), and this is combined, as already mentioned. as previously said, with specific strength and coordination exercises. You will observe how your fitness and mood will improve little by little. It is possibly the best investment in health you will make for yourself.

3. Recovery phase

In the last 5-10 minutes, it is imperative in cardiology patients to progressively reduce the intensity of the resistance phase until the resting situation. This gradual decrease will, in some cases, prevent the appearance of arrhythmias caused by the sudden stop of physical exercise and the appearance of other adverse effects such as dizziness or hypotension. Finally, stretching/flexibility exercises will be performed again to recover and relax muscle tone, with about 3 repetitions per muscle group and maintaining each stretch for 20-30 seconds.

CHAPTER FOUR

Easy-to-Follow Meal Preps: "I'm never consistent."

You've probably heard that meal planning is an excellent way to heal your finances. If your food expenses are high, and you often wonder, what can I cook today? You should definitely consider creating a meal list. I know it's hard to go from theory to practice because establishing a system and creating a meal plan will take a long time. When you want to implement something new, questions like these arise:

- Is it worth doing?

- What benefits will I get?

- Can I be successful at it?

There are many reasons why it is worth taking your time to create a meal plan. With careful organization, you know in advance what you need for each meal and have time to shop or defrost something if necessary. This way, you reduce the stress that cooking causes you, and the most important thing is that you can better control your food expenses.

Why do you need to plan your meals?

1. To save time.

Preparing the meal plan takes a little time, but the time you can save is much more. How often have you asked yourself: What will I cook this day? What will I prepare for dinner? With a plan in place, this dilemma no longer exists. Every time you start working right away. In addition, by having the list, you significantly shorten the time needed to make purchases.

2. To save money.

Meal planning helps you avoid impulse purchases. With a good shopping list, you only need one or two weekly visits to the store. In addition, it allows you to make better use of discounts, because you know the quantity and type of products you will need in the coming days.

3. To take care of your health.

Planning all your meals for the day will help you eat healthier. You will avoid going for fast foods, most of which contain preservatives and other harmful ingredients. Homemade food from fresh ingredients is the most beneficial solution. I think "by taking care of healthy eating – you don't waste your money on doctors."

How to start meal planning?

1. Make a list of 15-20 of your favorite foods

To make this list, sit down with your entire family and ask everyone about their favorite foods. Once this is done, look at the list and select those meals that are quick and easy to prepare and don't need too many ingredients. The best if they are healthy meals.

2. Gather the recipes for the meals you are going to prepare

Organize your list. You can divide meals into groups, for example, soups, meat dishes, and vegetarian dishes, so they are easy to manage.

Find the recipes you need and write them down or print them on sheets of paper. Also, you can consider purchasing a special notebook for recipes. The most important thing is easy access to them because you will need them often.

3. Plan meals for the entire day

Don't limit yourself to just creating a lunch list. Eating 3-5 times a day is advisable, so think about planning all your breakfasts, lunches and dinners.

4. Write your menu on paper

You have many ways to do it. Personally, I use the "weekly meal plan" template. It's where I write my menu for the entire week and then print it. Another way is to use a notebook. On the left side of the page, you write a list of your meals; on the right side, write all the ingredients necessary to prepare this meal (in one go, you will have a meal plan and shopping list). Regardless of your chosen method, make your plan visible to everyone in the house. The best place is the kitchen.

5. Check what you have in your pantry

Before putting your menu into action, it's a good idea to check your pantry, refrigerator and freezer. Organize all the food you have there: throw away what is already expired, and organize everything else into appropriate groups (see the shopping list template for an example of groups)

6. Adjust the menu according to your family's eventualities

When you're planning meals, take into account your daily activities and those of your family. Did your children eat lunch at school? Plan a more modest lunch at home that day.

Are you coming home late from work? Think about a dinner that takes a little time to prepare. Has the family been invited to a Sunday dinner? You don't have to prepare dinner that day. It is good to consider all the related factors and consider them when creating your menu.

7. Use seasonal products

Depending on the season, the availability of individual fruits and vegetables can change dramatically. Therefore, their prices also change. The best prices will be found during the harvest, resulting in savings.

The point is that it is expected that your menu can change during the year. I recommend using fresh seasonal ingredients from your garden or those available in the market at this time of year.

8. Prepare more meals at once

Do you think about eating the same dish more than once a week? Try to prepare a larger quantity of this meal for today and the next few days. If you do, put the separated food into containers and place them in the refrigerator or freezer. You can also bottle the food in jars.

9. Plan your food "cleanse" day

If you collect all the leftover food from your refrigerator at the end of the week, you can plan a night when you and your family have only the leftovers for dinner. That day, you should also check which products are close to the expiration date and which are the products to use in meals for the next few days.

10.   Review your daily plan

Your meal plan should be flexible. If necessary, don't be afraid to make modifications and use opportunities. Imagine that on the way home, you notice a promotion for your favorite fish. You buy this fish, prepare a fillet, and the lunch planned for today is postponed until the next day. Remember that this plan should be tailored to you, not you to it.

Weekly menus with careful planning enable us to follow the World Health Organization's recommendations, which suggest including fruits and vegetables, proteins, and carbohydrates in every meal. We'll eat better, reduce our money on food, and free up time and responsibilities.

CONCLUSION

Celebrating success is an essential part of our path to achieving our goals and aspirations. It allows us to recognize our achievements, reflect on the hard work and effort invested, and find motivation to strive for greatness. For example, our goal is to lose weight, celebrating every pound lost or fitness milestone reached can motivate us toward our overall goal.

Overcoming obstacles requires perseverance and a positive mindset. Stay motivated by remembering your goals and why you started on this path in the first place. Surround yourself with positive influences and participate in activities that inspire and encourage you.

Fitness is a physical activity focused on the progressive improvement of muscle tone. Combining its practice with an adequate diet is fundamental to good health. Apart from weight loss, we must add the improvement of cardiovascular health. Remember that a balanced diet must go hand in hand with your fitness session. People with a positive energy balance had an increase in daily energy expenditure, meaning their bodies burned more calories overall compared to those with a negative energy balance.

Creating and maintaining a positive energy balance through proper nutrition and exercise is critical to achieving optimal health and fitness.

Continuing to follow the tips in this guide will improve your health and increase your chances of achieving your weight loss goal. Remember, consistency is key!

www.ingramcontent.com/pod-product-compliance
Lightning Source LLC
Chambersburg PA
CBHW051728250726
48653CB00008B/3259